Eat Like A White Chick

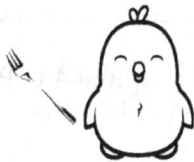

Norma G. Jackson

Eat Like A White Chick

Published by Inspired 4 U Publications
www.howtoselfpublishinexcellence.com

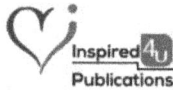

Statistic Sources: WebMD, SELF Magazine, and Women Enews

ISBN-13: 978-0-9994252-0-6
ISBN-10: 099942520X

Dedication

Usually, a book dedication gives credit to the wind beneath the wings of an author. I can't do that because I don't even know the name of the person I met at an airport who inspired me to write my story. Wherever she is, I hope one day she will read this book and get in touch with me. I would give her the true thanks she is due.

My brief encounter with a blonde traveler began as we both placed our luggage down in an airport café in Dallas. We joked about mounting the high stools at the counter. I said something funny about having to really 'hoist it up there' with my 5'10" 300+ lb frame. She was shorter and smaller framed, but not skinny. As we chatted about the weather, she opened up more. She probably thought, "I'm just having a brief conversation during a layover." However, what happened next was quite remarkable. Our conversation turned to food as soon as our orders arrived. Now that I was no longer a stranger, she felt free to assess my plate and offer some friendly advice.

"You know, I love sandwiches too, but

bread holds a lot of water and makes me feel so bloated after I eat it. One trick I discovered is to remove the spongy part of the bread from the inside of the bun, and keep the remaining bread to cover the top and bottom of my sandwich. It has fewer calories and causes less bloating. I feel like I'm still eating a sandwich and I don't even miss the spongy part." As she spoke, I was intrigued by her obvious joy in this discovery.

For most of you reading this, that may have been a "duh" moment; but for me, it was a real transformative "AHA" moment. I thought: *What else do you know that I don't? Are there other techniques that I could learn and copy to benefit my health?*

In that moment, I recounted my personal journey with food and decided that this Black Chick was going to "Eat Like A White Chick" (ELAWC) from now on.

TABLE OF CONTENTS

My vision is to wake up my African-American sisters
and break the yoke of sickness.

INTRODUCTION

"Eat Like A White Chick" is intentionally meant to be provocative. My vision is to wake up my African-American sisters collectively and break the yoke of sickness, lifetime medications, poor choices and unhealthy habits. I recognize this may be challenging to do and that I walk a thin line in the delivery of my message, but...

I pray that you will hear my heart and know that it is not my intention to offend those of you who are doing the right thing for your health or to imply that all white chicks eat healthy and all black women don't.

The true intent of my book is love. It is love for black women and love for myself, and it is encouragement to do better as we know better. We as black women have counted on the government to subsidize our bad choices, but that train is coming to the end of the station.

I believe success leaves clues that you can study and apply to achieve the same results.

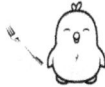

EAT LIKE A WHITE CHICK?

Say What? Eat Like A White Chick? Huh? Yep, that's what I decided. Yes, I'm totally sane with a bold message and I've heard that once you find something you're passionate about, you will want to share it.

This book will not be viewed as 'middle of the road' advice. You will either love or despise the fact that I strongly agree with the Shakespearean quote that states, "The fault lies not in our stars, but in ourselves." And I invite you to put aside all of your negative stereotypes about how white women eat and secretly *un-eat*. We are going to look closely at the positive behaviors only, and incorporate them in our routine.

This is also an invitation to the white chick, who isn't really eating like a white chick as described in this book, to climb on board and ride alongside us.

I encourage you to unashamedly admit today that perhaps you could learn something by eating like a white chick. In other words, we eat differently than white chicks, and therefore have different results in our health. Some could say, "We eat differently than Asians also, so why are you just talking about white women?" I'm just talking about white women because the images I'm bombarded with on TV, movies and the stage of what the American woman's body shape should look like usually comes in a steady stream of white chick images.

During my professional life in sales, I always looked for a mentor because I didn't believe in recreating the wheel. I learned from success coach Tony Robbins that success leaves clues that you can study and apply to achieve the same results. So when it came to finding a mentor who had successfully navigated the field of food, I looked to those who were healthier than me.

Just hear me out without looking for

excuses to disagree. We (African-American women) are AWESOME to our cores! In general, we are the backbone, the glue, or whatever you want to call it, that keeps things going. We bend, but don't break under pressure, and still we rise! I could go on and on; however, we need to kill the idea that we are somehow winning the race to a healthier relationship with food, because we aren't. We are going in the wrong direction. Like the death of so many ideas, in the aftermath there comes DENIAL, GUILT, and finally ACCEPTANCE.

To smack the face of DENIAL, here are the statistics from WomensHealth.Gov and they ain't pretty:

Health conditions common in African-American women– Of all minority groups, African-Americans have the majority of health conditions and most of the time, the greatest differences in health risks when compared to others. African-Americans also have more early deaths, disabilities, and diseases. Google any source and you'll find that the top health concerns facing African-American women are consistent with the list on the next page. Many of these problems are chronic, which means they last a long time and sometimes forever. However, many of these problems can also be prevented.

- ✓ Asthma
- ✓ Breast cancer
- ✓ Cancer
- ✓ Cervical cancer
- ✓ Diabetes
- ✓ Glaucoma and cataracts
- ✓ Heart disease
- ✓ High blood pressure
- ✓ High cholesterol
- ✓ HIV/AIDS
- ✓ Infant death
- ✓ Kidney disease
- ✓ Lupus
- ✓ Osteoporosis
- ✓ Overweight and obesity
- ✓ Pregnancy-related death
- ✓ Sexually transmitted infections (STIs)
- ✓ Sickle cell anemia
- ✓ Smoking
- ✓ Stroke
- ✓ Tuberculosis (TB)
- ✓ Uterine fibroids
- ✓ Violence

Enough said? This, by the way, is a short

Googled list of ailments that affect African-American women. Whatever the reasons are for this health gap, African-American women can take charge of their personal health and empower themselves.

I can hear you saying, "Lack of healthcare plays a large part in some of these issues." This is true. The fact is that African-American women are less likely to receive healthcare and when they do get care, they are more likely to get it too late. For instance, problems like breast and cervical cancer aren't found early when they are most treatable; and the chance to prevent or delay diabetes is often lost. Generations of racism and poverty also play a part. There is also lack of trust in the medical system, cultural differences, obstacles accessing care, and a lack of knowledge about the importance of screening for major health problems. Similarly, genetics contribute to the risk in some cases. The reasons are numerous.

If you've been paying attention to the healthcare landscape in America, you'll agree that now, more than ever, is the time that we must take charge of our own health. The government will be cutting back on care for the obese, the chronically ill, and the poor and sick Americans, in general. The sick will be escorted to state-run high risk pools, which will prove to be as expensive as it sounds.

As I'm writing, CNBC News just announced that "One-half of all black women are obese in America." Now that's a statistic to contemplate for now and the future. Some scientists say black women lack the gene that tells us we are satisfied when we eat. The reason for that is because when our enslaved ancestors were made to work 14-hour days picking cotton, they never knew where their next meal was coming from. It was probably a combination of 'when and where'. So to adapt, their bodies turned off the normal gene that would signal 'they've had enough'. They had to hoard energy for later use, like squirrels hoarding nuts for the winter. I don't know if that is a viable reason that contributes to the problem, but whatever the reason, we can only concentrate on things we can control. And I dare say that our ancestors would much prefer for us to focus on being victors instead of victims.

So while I wrote this book in a tongue-in-cheek style, my primary objective is to cajole, entertain and infuriate my *Sisters* into *doing something different*. Why? Because we all know that to do the same thing over and over (i.e., drinking diet sodas for breakfast) and expect a different outcome, like good health, is 'cray-cray'.

Now open your minds, chuckle if you like, and by all means, adopt a few of the suggestions offered in ELAWC.

Better health to us all!

Although black don't crack on the outside, we are starving our internal organs of water.

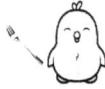

THEIR LOVE AFFAIR WITH WATER

Put down your Diet Coke for a minute and ponder this. It's been said that "Black don't crack" and it's true. Women of color have some of the most beautiful skin tones on the planet, but here's a thought: *What if we cherished water like a white chick?* Meaning, we never leave home without it. We would sip water in the car, in the gym, during the meeting, on the toilet. We would even keep water on our nightstands to welcome us to the morning light. Imagine if we chose to never be seen in public without water by our side? And to all of you waitresses who try to shame us by asking, "What will you be drinking besides water?" Our answer is, "NOTHING!"

We need to take serious note. White chicks have gadgets on their sleeves, on their bikes, in their cars, and on their babies' strollers that are all designed to hold water close to them. While we're clipping coupons for the next BIG GULP, white chicks are flushing out toxins and hydrating trillions of cells. Although black don't crack on the outside, we are starving our internal organs of water.

I'm not talking to those of you who love water. This is for those of you like me, who can't stand water. If you think or feel like you'd rather die of thirst than drink water, this next section is especially for you.

What can water do that Slurpees can't? Water lubricates our tissues and organs. Our eyes, brains and spinal columns are protected by the lubricating effects of water. Water aids in our digestion and replenishes saliva and digestive juices. The water in our body also helps to lubricate our joints.

In the black community, we always joke about 'Arthur Itis' who pays us a visit in old age and makes it painfully difficult to climb steps, put on shoes, or go for walks. Why don't we fight *Arthur* by drinking more water instead? Then we'd be proactively taking preventive measures to avoid becoming victims of *Mr. Itis*. Fruits and vegetables also kill the inflammation caused by this destroyer of good health.

When we drink adequate water, our body temperature is regulated through perspiration. The absence of sufficient water intake to replace the fluids we lose via sweat, respiration, tears and body waste can keep our bodies from perspiring enough to regulate our internal temperature. We often joke about our menopausal *personal summers* as we sweat like 'oink oinks'; but if we drank more water, could we possibly control the seasons and enjoy a refreshing Springtime or brisk Fall instead?

You ask, "What about the taste of water (or lack thereof)?" Well, if we can turn pig knuckles, pig feet, pig tails, intestines and snouts into fabulous fare, surely we are creative enough to flavor water and make it palatable. In fact, there are already several flavored and sparkling water options on the market. Don't you agree? So let's summon the same innate talent and power of choice to hydrate ourselves, our minds, and our bodies with water.

If we make poor food choices, our children are more likely to follow in that unhealthy lifestyle.

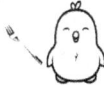

OUR FOOD CHOICES MATTER

We shout in protest that "Black Lives Matter" while we cut our own lives short with bad food choices. Which do you consider is the worse scenario?

1) What others do to us?
2) What we do to ourselves?

This is what we do:

- **Sausage and Pancakes**

We are stuck and unimaginative when it comes to what we eat for breakfast. White chicks break their fast with literally anything healthy. They will eat a vegetable salad with boiled eggs and quinoa for breakfast. Other choices may be fruit and cottage cheese or leftover baked chicken and a handful of walnuts. What? That doesn't sound like breakfast to you? Do like the catch-phrase in the 1971 Alka-Seltzer commercial suggests, "Try it, you'll like it!"

- **Fried Dyed and Laid to the Side**

No, I'm not talking about your hair, but I got your attention, didn't I? I'm talking about the fried oil baptisms that we give our meals. Baked, stewed, and braised are not bad words. They are just better alternatives to preparing healthier food.

- **Food as a Friend vs. Fuel**

While our salivary glands swell when we think of comfort food, white chicks believe food is to be used as fuel for the body. They know that using food as a friend to try and fill the hole inside when you're hurting does not work. Your man left you.... So what? Take it out on him, not your body. Ask yourself, "Am I hungry or do I want to kill somebody?"

White chicks will grab their tennis shoes

and go for a walk or run before they sabotage their bodies.

- ## The Ripple Effect

Generations are affected by the examples we set. Our children follow what we do more than what we say. If we make poor food choices, our children are more likely to follow in that unhealthy lifestyle.

I choose not to take my granddaughter to fast food places. As a result, she loves quinoa and black bean soup; and she likes cut veggies and fresh fruit.

- ## Undervalue Ourselves

What in this society tells a black woman she is valuable, loveable and deserving of honor? We are often portrayed as 'angry black women'. Do we have reasons to be angry? Yes, we do. But by focusing on those reasons we miss the point. We get angry and return to the "Watts" mentality of burning down our own cities and stores; or in this case, we destroy our own bodies and health, one bag of french fries at a time.

Oprah had it right when she said, "Focus on what you are grateful for." Futhermore, if you must be angry, be angry that far too many of us don't treat our bodies like a temple. We can be found every Sunday in a house of worship, but the second most important commandment to "Love your neighbor as yourself" is a lesson some of us miss.

As a child, my mother told me stories of how she was treated during the war effort in the 40's. She had a college degree, typed 80 wpm, and took shorthand at 140 wpm. She stood in line to get a government job behind a white woman who had a high school degree, typed 40 wpm, and didn't know how to take dictation. My mother watched as the woman without skills was offered a secretarial job while she was offered a position in the factory making ammunition.

Was it fair? Not in the least. But instead of being consumed with bitterness, my mother taught us thankfulness. For instance, if you complained that you got a bonus of $500 only to discover that you owed a $499 bill, she would always say,

"Just be thankful that you had the money to pay it." Hearing that advice would drive me crazy. But now that I'm older, I see the wisdom in being grateful. In fact, I'm simply grateful just to be alive.

I have eaten for sheer pleasure throughout my life,
until the consequences caught up to me as an adult and
squeezed out my joy of eating.

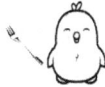

MY STORY

A Fun-Loving Childhood

In 1957, I was the product of two wonderful parents, Myrtice Murray and Norman Willis Goodwin. I was named Norma Wyllis Goodwin, after dad, and my older brother Emerson Murray Goodwin (Em) shared mom's maiden name. Our parents had their two children late in life. You could probably say we were raised by 'grandparent-like' parents.

Em and I came on the scene after our parents had been married for 14 and 16 years, respectively. For years, their friends kept telling them to settle down and have some kids; but for these two major league bridge players, settling down wasn't on the scorecard. I heard tales of their weekend escapades. They would come home from work, take two nose dives of Old Grand Dad whiskey, and start playing round-robin games of bridge and pinochle. They and their friends formed teams and, in-between games, each team would take turns sleeping on the couch. They would play non-stop through the weekend, from Friday until the wee hours of Monday morning. Then, they would take a shower and go to work.

My parents had fast and furious fun, and they loved life. Their fun and love of life was showered on me and Emerson like rain on flowering seeds. It made us feel truly wanted, special, and appreciated. They laughed hard, worked hard, and let us know we could do anything we set our minds to do. Emerson and I assumed that all families laughed and loved like ours. To this day, Em and I can make each other laugh so hard that we can only throw our heads back and roll from side to side without making a sound because we can barely breathe. It's that kind of laughter that feels like it could kill you if it lasted a minute longer. Even though Em was slender and I was not, he never kidded me about my weight. He was, and still is to this day, the epitome of what a big brother should be– *A Protector.*

Who knows why Em didn't cut my life short when we were children. I ate anything he put in the refrigerator for himself. Time after time, he would return to the fridge expecting to see that ham sandwich or whatever. It wasn't until he put cigarette butts in his soda can, as a special treat for me, did I change my ways.

Eating Habits and New Experiences

Emerson and I were both underweight babies of 5 lbs. He grew up tall and thin while I grew up a chubby baby, first grader, and teen. In the fifties, there weren't many warnings about drinking during pregnancy and mom enjoyed a martini as part of her daily routine. Maybe that explains our weird sense of humor, the kind of humor that can find funny in anything.

Most of my eating habits were molded by the cooking styles of Madison, GA and Greenville, SC, which were the birthplaces of mom and dad. What shape did that take on my plate? Lots of brown and white that consisted of fried chicken, fried pork chops, french fries, rice and potatoes. On Friday evenings, we ate vegetables, spaghetti, and fried perch, even though Daddy wasn't a Catholic. I guess he thought his family should be compliant to fish on Fridays just in case it had any spiritual merit. Sunday's breakfast included Polish Kielbasa sausage, Jimmy Dean sausage patties, thick bacon slices, scrambled eggs, cheesy grits, fried green tomatoes, buttered biscuits, and yes, the rice. We had to have rice because Emerson hated grits. *'Go figure.' And with southern parents?!* Did I mention a fruit we ate regularly? I think it was grapefruit with ½ an inch of sugar mounded on top. We were meat heavy and veggie lean.

I first learned some regional and cultural differences in food when I was in the 11th grade while participating in an orchestral exchange program. The program paired two students from different schools for a two week time period. My family hosted a white teenage girl from Massachusetts and subjected her to the breakfast I described earlier. She lived with us in Maryland for a week and performed two joint concerts at our high school. After the week was over, it was my turn to meet her parents and live with her in Massachusetts performing the same clarinet pieces in her hometown high school orchestra.

For breakfast I ate lochs and bagels with cream cheese. I wished for bacon and eggs, but that didn't make it so. Maybe I was too far north. I distinctly recall the huge smile on my exchange student's face after the southern breakfast. I also had a smile on my face after eating the lochs. Although different, they were good. I was very thankful for such cultural exchanges. Even more than the joint musical concerts we performed, I was grateful for the mutually enriching joint living experience and exchange of ideas.

Along with pleasant childhood memories of new experiences and eating my favorite foods, I also have nauseating memories of visits to Lane Bryant with my mother. At a young age, I realized that there was a special section for kids my size. The bottom line is that throughout my life, I ate for sheer pleasure until the consequences caught up to me as an adult and squeezed out my joy of eating.

The Diagnosis and Discovery

In October of 2006, I walked out to my mailbox at the end of my driveway and realized the air in my lungs was also at its end. My breathing was labored and I felt slightly dizzy. In an attempt to shrug it off, I thought— *Maybe I'll stop by the health clinic after I make a run to the dry cleaners.* But by the time I backed out of the driveway, my priorities had shifted. Still out of breath, I decided a stop by the clinic should come first. That was a good decision. What happened next came in such rapid succession. White coats surrounded me in my curtained off emergency room. I was repeatedly told the expected time of arrival for the ambulance and that I would soon be taking a trip to the hospital for cardiac tests.

While trying to digest that news, I was informed of a startling diagnosis. "Ms. Jackson, did you know that you are a diabetic?" My answer was, "No." But, should I have suspected? Probably.

My father was on insulin and my mother was taking some pills called Glucophage. At the time, I didn't know what the pills my mother took were for. We lived by the code of silence in our home when it came to health. As a family, we would talk about anything and everything, except our health or medicine. The idea that children might benefit from knowing what diseases run in the family was a foreign one. It wasn't until I was in my forties that I learned if one parent has diabetes, their child has a 50% chance of getting it. If you have two parents with diabetes, their child has an 80% chance of developing the disease. Had I known this in grade school, I probably would have spit out the candy "Now or Laters" immediately.

So off I went for further tests, whisked away to the nearest hospital by ambulance with a deafening siren. Results? One blocked artery. But because it wasn't a major artery, diet and exercise were prescribed. However, that diagnosis was severely challenged less than a week later.

I was about an hour from home when I suffered a flat tire. Fortunately, I was able to get to an auto garage quickly. I recounted my tire dilemma to the four guys I saw sitting in the garage bay doing nothing. Almost in unison, they explained how it was close to 5 p.m. on a Friday and they were no longer on the clock. Apparently, there would be no help coming my way from these four able-bodied men. It must have been the look of disbelief on my face, mourning the death of chivalry, or the look of utter desperation that led one of them to offer, "Meineke is around the corner. They might be able to help you."

If I wasn't a tooth grinder before that moment, I became one after it. Surely, the steam coming out of my ears was visible to my four faux automotive friends. Temper smoldering, I reluctantly got back in my car and limped on three good tires towards the Meineke shop around the corner. However, before I could make it to the entrance, my right hand instinctively clenched my chest and my eyes bulged with the realization of what my brain had assessed: *Yes, I am having an angina attack!* The pain was insufferable and not at all funny like Fred Sanford's depictions, on the old "Sanford & Son" sitcom, of having the 'BIG One'.

My calmer-self posed a logical question, "Where are those nitro tablets you were given in case something like this ever happened?" Rumbling in my purse, racing against time, I finally fumbled my fingers in place to open the bottle. After taking two sublingual tablets and waiting the required time period without relief, I anxiously read the instructions again.

"If after taking 3 pills you achieve no relief, immediately call 911." I inserted the third, tiny nitro pill under my tongue and prayed. Within a few seconds, I was grateful for the ability to take deep breaths again. Those pills saved my life.

Next, I needed to speak with the cardiologist who had prescribed them. It was a brief call. I described that I almost died, and he explained how I shouldn't have because it was only one blockage and not a main artery. *Anywho*, we did agree that I needed to be seen immediately for a balloon angioplasty to enlarge the artery, and that I also needed a medicated stent placed to keep it open, as the following step.

On the day of the surgery, I felt psyched because I had read that it was a common procedure. They would use a catheter with a camera and perform the whole operation through my groin. It was not without risks, but then again, no surgery is. Besides, after the valium pills, I felt like a party was going on. I was also given Demerol to put me in another world.

All was going well, and I was feeling no pain until the time came to insert the stent. How do I know the exact moment? It was when I began to experience the pain of a collapsing arterial wall that was being flattened by a stent. I started to moan and move on the operating table, trying to speak. I was basically saying, "You're killing me," in *demerolese*. The doctor knew exactly what I was saying and calmly explained that he caused the pain while placing the stent. This did nothing to boost my confidence and what followed later did even less.

I heard my cardiologist curse out loud in shock and say, "It seems we have two blocked arteries behind each other instead of one. What are we going to do?" Now I can't tell you the thoughts that go through your head when you're on an operating table and realize that the one operating is facing a situation he's never experienced before and is completely lost. We were both lost, but I was the one with my life in his hands.

The more I thought about my medical predicament, the more I moaned louder and louder. Then I heard a second voice that seemed to echo in the operating room. The voice belonged to a younger man, who sounded calm and surprisingly more experienced. It's almost as if he had been observing the operation up to this point and was now stepping in to lend his expertise. He said, "We will implant two stents. One will be kissing the other in the shape of a V."

I don't know who was more relieved, me or the senior operating cardiologist. We both exhaled, and then he realized what he needed to do. The last thing I heard before the anesthesia kicked in was his loud order, "Give her more Demerol! I want her completely out!" I didn't remember anything for days after that. The two stents were in place and the warning from the cardiologist was friendly, but stern. He said, "Had we known you had 2 blocked arteries (one 85% and the other 95%) we wouldn't have used a 'cath' procedure. The second blocked artery didn't show on the MRI. It was the ultrasound on the operating table that discovered it. Had we known, we would have had to break your ribs and perform open heart surgery. You're only 48 and way too young for open heart surgery." Then, with a warm smile he added, "Please, keep me out of your chest."

Well, it's been a total of 11 years clear since that harrowing incident with the stents in 2006. I've done my best to keep my cardiologist out of my chest. However, diabetes, the other disease they discovered, is a challenge I'm still fighting daily.

Diabetes

Diabetes runs rampant in the African-American community. Many of us have made it a habit to over-tax our pancreas with sugar-laden fare and overload our bodies with carbohydrates.

What about the white chick and diabetes? Here are the facts:

- The prevalence of diabetes is at least 2 to 4 times higher among African-American, Hispanic/Latino, American-Indian, and Asian/Pacific Islander women than among white women.

- Over 11 million women in the US have diabetes.

- Women minorities are the hardest hit by type 2 diabetes.

- Because minority populations are expected to grow at a faster rate than the U.S. population as a whole, the number of women in these groups who are diagnosed with diabetes will increase significantly in the coming years.

At age 48, I tried fat-free diets with artificial sweeteners only to see the scale go up to 305 lbs. That's when it dawned on me that the money wasn't in dead or healthy people. The pharmaceutical companies make most of their money in keeping us as sick as possible. Does the government deserve some of the blame? Well, I think it's highly suspect that they still publish brochures with a pyramid eating plan that recommends 9 to 11 daily servings of grains. We can almost invert that pyramid to eat in the opposite manner of what is recommended and improve our health. Yes, eat more fruits and vegetables, fewer grains, less dairy, and eat more high quality protein, nuts and seeds. Is this radical thinking? Yes, it is!

If you can't boil water, learn the art of preparing dishes that taste good and are good for you.

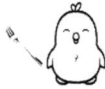

THE SOUL 30 PLAN

There has been a recent trend in radical eating plans. The Whole 30 diet plan emphasizes eating more whole foods, less processed foods, and less sugar for 30 days. Experts say that it only takes 21 days to form a habit.

For our purposes, let's think of it as the 'Soul 30 Plan' to improve our health. For 30 days, women of color can enlist the aid of good friends and agree to eat as close to the earth as possible. This means if it hangs from a tree or pushes up from the ground, we can eat it. If it's in a box or a bag and has more than five (5) ingredients, think twice before ingesting. In doing so, we will breathe life and rainbow colors into our dishes with fresh or raw foods. If you can't boil water, learn the art of preparing dishes that taste good and are good for you. Google recipes and watch videos that teach you how to prepare food. Allrecipes.com is a great place to start.

Eight Winning Strategies

Engage in the following strategies to help you succeed in your journey:

1. **Crawl Before You Walk**

   We know that sweet drinks are hard to give up, so crawl before you walk. Fill your glass with ¼ cup of sweet tea and ¾ cup of unsweetened tea. Eventually, you can go cold turkey and jump right into unsweetened tea. Do the same with fruit juices- ¼ juice and ¾ water, seltzer or Perrier. We aren't looking for perfection, just a reduction of sugar.

2. **Farewell to Fast Food Addiction**

   Do the fast food drive-thru workers all know you by name? When they say good-bye, do they quickly follow it up with, "See you tomorrow?" If so, then you may have a fast food addiction. Try the trick I learned at the beginning of my journey. Remove the huge spongy top lid from any sandwich and throw it into the wind. Feel good about feeding the birds, ants or whatever.

Also, do fries always have to go with the sandwich? Can't we choose a salad or another side? Yes we can!

3. **A Small Plate**

If you start with a smaller plate, you can go back for seconds and still eat less food than you are accustomed to. Put away the dishes that really hold three servings of spaghetti with room to spare. They are way too big. When *Shaq comes over for dinner, you can pull them out again.

Shaq (Shaquille O'Neal, Basketball Star)

4. **Plate it Right**

If you fill up 2/3 of your plate with veggies first, you will have crowded out the space for anything other than a fist-sized portion of meat and some fruit. Let's plate it right!

5. **Cut the Carbs**

If you must have the beloved Mac n Cheese or the mashed potatoes, make it ¼ cup. I know we've been taught that ½ cup is good, but we can do better.

6. **Get Fit**

My daughter bought me a FitBit. It actually tells me when I'm being sedentary and sends me an encouraging message to get up and move. Let's get up and go. Take a 10 minute walk with a work buddy on your break. Joining a gym is a great goal, but to crawl first just get moving and continue to add steps to your day. It can even be as minimal as stepping from side-to-side while you brush your teeth in the morning.

My Fitbit makes me WANT to park further away from the grocery store so I can accumulate extra steps during my day. Joining challenges to compete with friends and family, who also have a FitBit, is another fun way to stay motivated and keep moving.

7. **Let's Dance**

It's in our culture and DNA to dance. We celebrate by dancing at barbecues, picnics, family reunions, and card parties.

Who said you need a lot of people around to dance? Let's dance when nobody is looking. It's okay to turn the music on and dance by yourself.

Will you commit to adding 15 minutes of dancing to your day or week?

8. **Stop the Process**

Surgeons with over 25 years experience and thousands of open heart surgeries are recently speaking out and admitting that they were wrong to believe that heart disease was caused by too much fat. Fat does not give you high cholesterol. Inflammation of your arteries will. What causes inflammation in your aterial wall?

The real culprit is too much sugar, and particularly processed foods. It seems those boxed processed helpers in the kitchen aren't helping us at all. The endless variety of chips we purchase and the bags of food handed out at the drive thru windows are processed to the max.

The cure? Stop the Process. In order to stay on a grocery store shelf day after day, the items must be processed. Shop the outer walls of the store for fruits, vegetables, nuts, seeds and lean meat – and leave the aisles of processed foods alone. Look in your shopping cart. Do you see cans of soda and processed fruit juices? Candy bars? Cakes, pies, cookies? Do you see boxes of food or actual food? Stop the process.

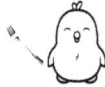

ACTIONS FOR TRANSFORMATION & THE SECRET

My goals for writing this book were to:

1. Get your attention
2. Involve your emotions
3. Educate, encourage and inspire
4. Motivate
5. Save a life

As I climb down from my provocative soapbox, I encourage you to stop using food as therapy. I know it's a scary thing to actually feel whatever pain you're facing in the moment instead of reaching for a chocolate bar or other comfort food. Asking yourself,

"What am I feeling and why am I feeling this way?" is a catalyst toward transformation. To ask is to realize that the plate of Mac n Cheese you want to consume is not going to change the moment for the better. To ask is to understand that the root problem will still be there after you eat it. In addition, you will also have the extra calories and additional pounds to contend with if you continue to make poor choices for emotional reasons.

Become self-aware by assessing where you are right now and determine where and how you want to be healthier in your life. Then use the suggestions in "Eat Like A White Chick" as a bridge to go from self-awareness to healthier choices.

Identify Your Why

No one takes action to solve a problem without having a big enough WHY. What is your "why"? List your top five reasons for wanting to be healthier below.

1. _____

2. _____

3. _____

4. _____

5. _____

Your five reasons should include YOU at the top in the number one spot. If your reasons are based on other people, an event or thing, then you have bought into the idea that you are not worthy. Think about it from the perspective of saving a life on an airplane. The flight attendant instructs you to place the oxygen mask on yourself first. Before you can help anyone else, you must begin within. All change begins with YOU.

Affirm Your Worthiness

Being worthy has been defined as "having enough good qualities to be considered important, useful, and deserving of respect, praise and attention." You are worthy despite how you were raised, despite what your best friend did, despite what men may have said and done to you, despite how your boss treats you, and despite your financial situation or how your children turned out. Despite anything you may have experienced of a negative nature up to this day, always remember that you are worthy!

Before you embark on this journey, I recommend the following exercise:

1. Affirm, out loud, one thousand times, "I am worthy of good health."

2. Set the timer for 15 minutes and go for it.

3. Listen for a difference in the tone of your voice. You will sound and feel more confident by the time you get to 100.

This is not some useless or stupid exercise to get through as quickly as possible. It is an effective way to re-program your mind with a strong message that we all need to hear and remember daily.

You are worthy and you deserve to be healthy. Once you put these suggestions into practice and start on your healthier journey, you will discover what you already knew before you started reading this book:

There is no need to *Eat Like A White Chick* or anyone else, for that matter. <u>The real secret</u> is to **"Eat Like You Are Worthy of Good Health,"** because you truly are!

**a Cheat Sheet for
Managing Chronic Disease**

Fight
Chronic Disease
& WIN!

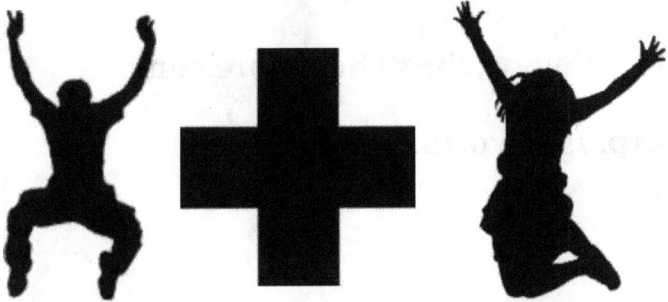

How to manage your IBS, diabetes, arthritis, psoriasis, hypertension or other chronic disease with healthy living and a healthy diet

Begin to Get Better Now!

I

Fight Chronic Disease and Win -How to manage your IBS, diabetes, arthritis, psoriasis, hypertension or other chronic disease with healthy living

ISBN: 1499732007
ISBN-13: 978-1499732009

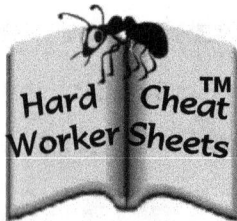

a *Hard Worker Cheat Sheet*™

for Better Health